HEALTH BENEFITS

OF

SOURSUP…

BY LAUCY KENNETH

"Did you know Soursop is 1000 times more effective than Chemotherapy?"

If you want to expand your mind with knowledge of a fruit you probably never knew existed, continue onward to see what soursop is and what it has to offer

COPYRIGHTS

HEALTH BENEFIT OF SOURSOP…written by Laucy Kenneth.

Compilation and cover design by:

D-xtreme Media LTD.

Direct copyright enquiries to:

Email: taddat@ymail.com

First published October 2014.

TABLE OF CONTENT

WHAT IS SOURSOP?

Soursop also known as 'Guyabano' is a fruit that comes from the Graviola tree. Other names for soursop :

Pawpaw (in Brazil),

guanábana (Spanish),

Africa and Southeast Asia

graviola (Portuguese),

guyabano (Philippines),

and custard apple (English).

The scientific name is annona muricata. The graviola tree grows in warm tropical areas such as the Philippines, South America, Africa and Southeast Asia. Known as a sedative, a nerve tonic, and used to maintain proper intestinal health, guyabano is just one medicinal tool stemming from the graviola tree. Throughout history, each part of the graviola tree, such as the bark, leaves, roots, fruit, and seeds have been used for medicinal purposes. The seeds have been used to treat nausea and vomiting, while herbal medicine practitioners recommend using the fruit and leaves to relieve stomach distress, pain, cough, asthma, and fever.A well-known fruit all over the world, the soursop's delicious white pulp, with tones of fruit candy and smooth cream is commonplace in tropical markets, but is rarely found fresh anywhere else. The graviola tree, or Annona muricata, produces the sweet soursop fruit, also called custard apple, paw paw or, in many Spanish-speaking countries, guanabana. The tree reaches a height of 25 or 30 feet and produces large fruit that may reach a length of 12 inchesInside its thin, leathery, green flesh is a large mass of creamy pulp, usually intermixed with 50-100 black seeds.

While the fruit is not as well known as others and is less researched, soursop health benefits are still worthy of note. soursop fruit is so delicious with a sharp aroma and a sweet-sour taste which is basically a combination of the taste of pineapple and strawberry. Recently, it has gained attention and popularity due to its natural cancer cell killing properties. There are also various uses of soursop apart from its anti- cancer properties. They have the Acetoginin containing compounds namely bulatacin, asimisin and squamosin. Acetoginin acts as an anti-feedent. Thus, they are often used in killing insects and pests which die by consuming these leaves even in small amounts. Scientific research conducted by The National Cancer Institute has proved that Soursop leaves can effectively attack and destroy cancer cells. In addition to this, they are also used in the treatment of several other diseases. Thus, the leaves have excellent medicinal properties making them usable as an ingredient in several herbal health products, they are rich in several compounds including protein, calcium, fructose, fat, vitamins A and B and the like. SOURSOP fruit, leaves and seeds, are useful as a natural remedy to treat a variety of diseases including Cancer, Lumbago, Ulcers, and Bladder Pain.

Guyabano (soursop) has been scientifically and traditionally proven to have great natural benefits. It helps lower fever, spasms, heart rate, and blood pressure. It also helps relieve pain, inflammation, and asthma. Consuming guyabano extract can also safely prevent cancer cells from forming while effectively slowing down tumor growth. It also helps stop the growth of harmful bacteria, viruses, fungi, and parasites, even as it stimulates digestion and stop convulsions.

Lifestyle and Cancer:

Cancer is not a disease whose origin is principally genetic, as many people continue to believe. It is a pathology that is closely linked to a range of lifestyle factors, particularly smoking and obesity (which stems from our sedentary habits and our dietary choices). Several studies have shown a direct link between the regular consumption of certain fruits and vegetables and a reduction in risk of developing various types of cancer.

HEALTH BENEFITS YOU WILL GET FROM SOURSOP FRUIT

1. Treatment and prevention of Cancer:

Unfortunately, research revolving around soursop's healing properties is lacking in the scientific world, but so far researchers have been studying soursop for its ability to protect against cancer and reduce side-effects of chemotherapy.

Since 1976, over 20 independent labs researched soursop's anti-cancer effects following initial research carried out by the National Cancer Institute. The National Cancer Institute found that soursop's "leaves and stems were found effective in attacking and destroying malignant cells. After the 1976 findings, that was apparently never released to the public, other research studies came out with similar conclusions:

- One study published in the Journal of Natural Products found that one chemical in Graviola was 10,000 times more potent than a chemotherapy drug called Adriamycin.

- The Catholic University of South Korea reports that guyabano is not only a threat to cancer cells, but also leaves healthy cells alone. This is not the case with chemo, which target all the cells – much like antibiotics indiscriminately destroying all gut bacteria, good and bad.

- Purdue University found that leaves from the guyabano tree are "killed cancer cells among six human cell lines". The researchers also found that the leaves were particularly effective for prostate and pancreatic cancers.

One piece of research found on PubMed concluded:

Overall, the compounds that are naturally present in a Graviola extract inhibited multiple signaling pathways that regulate metabolism, cell cycle, survival, and metastatic properties in PC cells. Collectively, alterations in these parameters led to a decrease in tumorigenicity and metastasis of orthotopically implanted pancreatic tumors, indicating promising characteristics of the natural product against this lethal disease."

While soursop has something to offer in the world of cancer protection, it's important to note that studies conducted with soursop were conducted in what's known as In Vitro. This means that biological component have been isolated for testing, and this this case, cancer cells were used in test tubes. While it's helpful to start research somewhere, we are still in need of human clinical trials. Soursop leaves can inhibit cancer cells and cure cancer more quickly and effectively than chemotherapy which results in several side effects besides being expensive. In fact, research has proved that soursop has an active ingredient that is 10000 times stronger than chemotherapy in fighting cancer cells. Thus, soursop leaves can treat different types of cancers including prostate, lung and breast cancers. For treatment, boil 10 soursop leaves in 3 cups of water until only one cup of water remains, strain and cool it and drink this concoction every morning for 3-4 weeks to determine improvement in the condition.

2. Treatment and prevention of urinary tract infections :

Soursop is known for its vitamin C content (77% daily value per cup). Vitamin C can help to decrease the amount of harmful bacteria that may be present in the urinary tract. In fact, many alternative medicines use soursop leaves for the treatment of gout. For this purpose, take 6 to 10 soursop leaves which are old but still green and wash them clean. Boil the leaves in 2 cups of water and simmer until one cup of water remains. This concoction should be taken twice a day i.e. morning and evening for maximum benefits. The soursop fruit has ascorbic acid which increases the amount of antioxidants in the body and also help keep a number of infections and disorders at bay.

3. Back Pain Treatment:

Back pain is commonly experienced these days, particularly while exercising. Using chemical drugs for back pain can cause side effects. Soursop leaves are an effective herbal remedy for treating back pain without any negative effect. For excellent performance, you can boil 20 pieces of soursop leaves in 5 cups of water until only 3 cups of water are left. You may drink ¾ cup of this concoction once in a day for relief.

4. Treatment of Rheumatism and skin problems

The flesh of the soursop is applied as a poultice unchanged for 3 days to alleviate eczema, rheumatism, skin eruptions and other skin problems to promote healing of wounds. Rheumatic diseases are commonly observed in elderly people, causing great pain. Soursop leaves are a natural treatment for arthritis pain. For this purpose, mashes the soursop leaves until they become smooth and apply on the areas of the body affected by pain due to arthritis regularly twice a day.

5. Treatment of Diabetes:

The limit of normal sugar levels ranges from 70 mg to 120 mg. The nutrients in soursop leaves are believed to stabilize blood sugar levels in the normal range. Besides, the extracts of soursop leaves can be used as one of the natural diabetes remedies. All this makes these leaves beneficial for diabetics.

6. Boosts the Immune System and Prevents Infections:

Along with vitamin C, soursop is known to be rich in B vitamins as well. B vitamins are known to help increase energy levels. The nutrient content of soursop leaves is believed to boost the immune system and avoid infections in the body. You may Boil 4/5 soursop leaves in 4 cups of water until one cup water remains and drink this concoction regularly once in a day for beneficial results.

7. Serves as antidote for poisoning and stomach troubles:

The seeds, which have emetic properties, can be used in the treatment of vomiting; Intestinal upset, stomach distress, prevention against constipation, the root bark is use as an antidote for poisoning. A decoction of the young shoots or leaves is regarded as a remedy for gall bladder trouble, diarrhea, dysentery, fever, indigestion as well as respiratory issues such as asthma or coughs, catarrh. In addition to the benefits mentioned above, soursop leaves are extremely effective in inhibiting the growth of bacteria, virus, parasites and tumor development. Their healing properties make them capable of being used as an anti-seizure medication. They help in treating inflammation and swollen feet. They aid in digestion and improve appetite. Soursop leaf consumption on a regular basis helps in improving stamina and facilitating quick recovery from diseases. Since the fruit contains soluble and insoluble fibers, it adds bulk to the stool and facilitates easy elimination from the body.

SKIN BENEFITS OF SOURSOP LEAVES:

Due to their medicinal properties soursop leaves are extremely beneficial for health. As pointed out earlier, they are used in the treatment of some of the deadliest diseases. The leaves offer some skin benefits as well.

8. Treatment of Boils:

Ulcer is a skin disorder that is characterized by immense pain and even has the risk of catching infection. Boils can occur on the body or on the face, thus interfering with your skin health and beauty. Soursop leaves are a natural remedy to cure ulcers. You can pick some young it leaves and place them on the body affected by ulcers.

9. Treatment of Eczema:

As already stated earlier, soursop leaves can treat eczema in a natural way. You can mash a few soursop leaves and apply it on the affected areas twice a day regularly. This will help in alleviating the pain caused by eczema besides treating it. A pulp made with fresh soursop leaves and rose water when applied on the skin can be very useful in preventing the occurrence of blackheads and other skin problems too.

10. Get rid of Head Lice and Bed Bugs

The use of soursop leaf decoction will not only get rid of pests but can also keep them away. All of us long for healthy and damage free hair. But unfortunately, the unhealthy lifestyle coupled with exposure to harmful chemicals and environmental pollutants is responsible for several hair problems like dandruff, split ends, hair loss, pre mature greying etc. Natural ingredients and herbal products can be very effective in combating these problems. As far as soursop leaves are concerned, much is not known about their benefits for hair. However, soursop leaves have the capability to inhibit the growth of parasites, besides other medicinal properties. Thus, applying a soursop leaf decoction on your hair can help you to get rid of head lice.

OTHER HEALTH BENEFITS OF SOURSOP INCLUDES

- ### Bone health –

    soursop contains copper, a mineral promoting the absorption of bone-benefiting calcium. Alleviates pain stemming from arthritis, joint and back problems, and rheumatism.

- ### Prevents leg cramps –

    Potassium in the fruit could help prevent leg cramps and also, decoction of leaves can be used as compresses for inflammation and swollen feet.

- ### Treat Mouth Ulcers–

    For real solution, finely mashing the leaf with water and applying it on the boils will help decrease the size of the ulcers in time curing them completely and also reduce irritation.

- **Prevention anemia and Kills Parasites –**

   Soursop (graviola) is rich in iron, which could help with iron deficiency anemia, it also Kills Parasites inside our Body as it is loaded with a number of nutrients essential for the overall development of body.

- **Migraine and headache relief–**

   Soursop (graviola) contains riboflavin, which could help with headaches and migraine relieve.

- **Reliever of liver ailment-**

   The juice of the fruit can be taken orally as a remedy for urethritis, haematuria and liver ailments. The juice when taken when fasting, it is believed to relieve liver ailments and leprosy.

RESEARCHES ON SOURPOP

Laboratory research supports the potential benefits of soursop as a remedy for disease. In one study, published in "Journal of Ethno pharmacology," an extract of soursop inhibited the growth of Herpes virus in the laboratory. In addition, the Cancer Center summarizes findings that suggest soursop extracts might slow growth of cancer cells or make them more susceptible to anti-cancer drugs. For example, in one study published in 1997 in "Journal of Medicinal Chemistry," compounds from soursop were tested on breast cancer cells in culture and found to be up to 250 times more effective in killing the cells than some chemotherapy drugs.

Researchers have revealed that a meal of soursop could be the cure for diabetes, heart disease, cancer, and diarrhea. Soursop is a medicinal plant that has been used as a natural remedy for a variety of illnesses. Several studies by different researchers demonstrated that the bark as well as the leaves has anti-hypertensive, vasodilator, anti-spasmodic (smooth muscle relaxant) and cardio depressant (slowing of heart rate) activities in animals.

Researchers had ascertained Soursop leaf's hypotensive (reduce blood pressure) properties in rats. Other properties and actions of Soursop documented by traditional uses include its use as anti-cancerous, anti-diabetes, anti-bacterial, anti-fungal, anti-malarial, anti-mutagenic (cellular protector), emetic (induce vomiting), anti-convulsant, sedative (induces sleep), insecticidal and uterine stimulant (helps in childbirth). It is also known to be a digestive stimulant, antiviral, cardio tonic (tones, balances and strengthens the heart), febrifuge (cures fever), nerviness (balances/calms the nerves), vermifuge (expels worms), pediculocide (kills lice) and as an analgesic (pain-reliever).

Researchers have confirmed the anti-viral activity of ethanolic extracts of Soursop against Herpes simplex virus. Extracts of Soursop have been shown to have anti-parasitic, anti-rheumatic, astringent, anti-leishmanial and cytotoxic effects. Soursop has also been shown to be effective against Multi-Drug Resistant (MDR) cancer cell lines. Extracts of Soursop were also shown to be effective against the cancer cell line U973, and hematoma cell lines in-vitro. Extracts were also shown to be lethal to the fresh water mollusk, Biomphalaria glabrata, which act as a host for the parasitic worm Schistosoma mansoni. But recent studies have described how extracts of Soursop reduces blood sugar in diabetics by improving insulin production, Improves cardiovascular health by reducing blood fats, treat drug resistant cancer, stop diarrhoea in children, among others.

COMPONENTS

Soursop contains a number of natural substances that have biological activity; these include fatty compounds called acetogenins, especially one called annonacin, along with other compounds called quinolones, annopentocins and two alkaloids, coreximine and reticuline. Soursop's acetogenins are the compounds that have been most studied, especially for their potential to prevent or slow the growth of cancer. The Cancer Center also says that some compounds in soursop may be naturally antiviral and anti parasitic, and may also suppress inflammation. Although its rind is quite bitter, the fruit's flesh is soft, smooth and sweet, and provides carbohydrate as its major nutrient. The fruit also contains abundant vitamin C and several B vitamins such as thiamin, riboflavin and niacin, along with calcium, phosphorus and a small amount of iron, but here is a fuller list of what the fruit has to offer:

- Riboflavin

- reticuline

- Phosphorus

- Acetogenins

- Vitamin and Iron

- Thiamine

- Calcium

- Carbohydrates

- Niacin

- Fiber

- Coreximine

- annonacin

OTHER IMPORTANT ANTI-CANCER FRUIT

Garlic

Several large studies have found that those who eat more garlic are less likely to develop various kinds of cancer, especially in digestive organs such as the esophagus, stomach, and colon. Ingredients in the pungent bulbs may keep cancer-causing substances in your body from working, or they may keep cancer cells from multiplying. The most powerful anti-cancer food was Garlic. Garlic stopped cancer growth completely against these tumor cell lines: Breast cancer, brain cancer, lung cancer, pancreatic cancer, prostate cancer, childhood brain cancer, and stomach cancer. Experts don't know how much you need to eat to prevent cancer, but a clove a day may be helpful.

Avocado

Avocado or alligator pear refers to the fruit of a tree native to Central Mexico. Botanically, it is a large berry that contains a single seed. The fruit may be pear-shaped, egg-shaped or spherical. Its name is taken from a Nahuatl word for "testicle".

Avocados contain lutein, an anti-cancer carotenoid. Lutein lowers the risk of prostate cancer in men and protects eyes against fatal diseases like macular degeneration and cataracts. Another cancer-fighting component of avocado is glutathione that can significantly cuts the incidence of oral and pharyngeal cancer. Avocados are also rich in potassium, vitamins, and heart-healthy fats.

Tomatoes

Some research has found that eating tomatoes may help protect men from prostate cancer. The juicy red orbs can help guard the DNA in your cells from damage that can lead to cancer. Tomatoes contain a particularly high concentration of an effective antioxidant called lycopene. Your body may absorb lycopene better from processed tomato foods such as sauce, which means that whole-wheat pasta with marinara sauce could be a delicious way to help lower your risk of this disease.

Pomegranate

The pomegranate is a berry and is between a lemon and a grapefruit in size, 5-12 cm in diameter. It has a rounded hexagonal shape and thick reddish skin. Native to Iran, the pomegranate has spread to Asian areas like the Caucasus and the Himalayas in Northern India.

Studies have reported that the fruits contain phytochemicals that can suppress aromatase, an enzyme which converts androgen into estrogen and which is associated with breast cancer. Furthermore, clinical trials have shown the pomegranate extracts can prevent prostate cancer in men.

IMPORTANCE OF THESE FRUITS:

It's particularly important to specifically include these in our diet, because not all fruits and vegetables share the same potential for active prevention against cancer. There are major differences in their levels of anticancer components. In some cases the phytochemical components that provide the greatest cancer-preventing activity are present only in a few, very specific fruits and vegetables. For example, the isoflavones of soy, the resveratrol of grapes, the curcumin of turmeric, the isothiocyanates and indoles of broccoli and the catechins of green tea are all anticancer molecules whose distribution among plants is extremely restricted.

In other words, even though all fruits and vegetables are an integral part of a balanced diet, only some of them can truly influence the risk of cancer.

DID YOU KNOW THAT EATING OF FRUITS CAN HELP YOU DIET AND LOSS SOME WEIGHT AND SHED UNNECESSARY FAT?

The secret shedding some weight falls on foods that contain water, like fruits and vegetables. *The consumption of fruit* provides *health benefits*, and so people who *take in* more *fruits* and vegetables as part of an overall healthy diet are likely to have a reduced risk of some chronic diseases. *Fruits* and vegetables are rich in vitamins and minerals that help you feel *healthy* and energized. *Healthy eating* includes *eating* at least five portions, and ideally 8 portions, of a different *fruits* or vegetables per day. According to the Center for Disease Control and Prevention 2009 statistics, 26.7 percent of adults in the U.S. are considered obese. This is a 9.6 percent increase from the year 2000. Given the prevalence of obesity, it is no surprise that Americans spend millions of dollars each year on losing weight. Weight loss is often achieved and maintained with multiple strategies among them we have: eating more fruits, vegetables and drinking of water.

Ever hear that water can help you lose a few extra pounds? It can if you eat foods that contain a lot of water, like fruits and veggies. In a University of Tokyo study, women who ate high-water-content foods had lower body mass indexes and smaller waistlines. Researchers speculate that the water in these foods may fill you up so you eat less. Make the strategy work for you by adding more of these in-season fruits and veggies—each is at least 90% water—to your meals. In this context, we will only be going through the act of eating fruits as this can help a greatly in dealing with stubborn fats in the body.

FRUIT FUNCTIONS

While fruit is naturally low in fat, sodium and calories, it is high in nutrients. Fruit contains abundant vitamins, fiber, antioxidants and potassium, all of which are important for optimal health. The U.S. Department of Agriculture's My Plate Food Guide recommends that adults consume 1.5 cups to 2 cups of fruit per day. Equivalents of one cup include one small apple, one large peach or orange, 32 grapes, one small wedge of watermelon or one cup of pineapple chunks.

Fiber:

Fruit is packed with fiber, an indigestible plant-based carbohydrate. Fiber adds bulk and volume without adding a lot of calories. Because of its bulk, fiber helps keep you full longer. A National Institute of Health newsletter reports that people on high fiber diets tend to eat about 10 percent fewer calories. In addition, other large studies found that people who have a high intake of fiber tend to weigh less. Fruit juice provides little or no fiber, so choose whole fruits. Eat the skins of fruits, such as apples, pears and peaches to maximize your fiber and vitamin benefits.

Low in Calories

Nutrient dense foods such as fruit provide a high amount of nutrients in a low calorie package. Fruit has high water content, contributing to satiety. Thirty-five overweight women were randomized to eat oat cookies, apples or pears three times per day along with a hypo caloric diet in a study from Maria Conceicao de Oliveira and team at the State University of Rio de Janeiro in Brazil. After 12 weeks, the fruit groups lost 1.21 kg compared to 0.88 kg in the oats group. However, the fruit groups had an increase in blood triglycerides at the follow-up.

Mixed Results

Replacing higher calorie and fat foods with fruit can aid in weight loss by decreasing your overall calorie intake. However, a more conventional low calorie diet outperformed a high fruit and vegetable diet in a study by Sherry Tanumihardjo and colleagues from the Department of Nutritional Sciences at the University of Wisconsin-Madison. In the study, some participants consumed a diet of eight servings per day of vegetables and two to three servings of fruit. The other group reduced caloric intake by 500 and consumed less than 25 percent of their calories from fat. At all three follow-ups -- three months, 12 months and 18 months -- caloric intake was significantly lower for the vegetable and fruit group, yet body mass index was lower only at the three month mark. At the 12 and 18 month marks, it was higher. The low-calorie, low-fat group had a lower body mass index at all three follow-ups.

Fructose

The mechanism by which fructose is metabolized in the liver may lead to an increase in blood triglycerides. The sweet sugar, fructose, is found naturally in fruit, vegetables and honey, or manufactured into high-fructose corn syrup. According to the International Food Information Council Foundation, one theory behind the role of fructose in obesity is that fructose does not affect the hormones that regulate hunger and food intake in the same way as other carbohydrates. The foundation notes that the speculation is based on research involving large amounts of fructose, three to four times the amount in the typical American diet.

CONCLUSION

It is thought that eating soursop or drinking the juice regularly may help prevent cancers. The leaves of the soursop, taken as a herbal infusion, are believed to help reduce cancerous cells in patients. Much like chemotherapy, the tea is thought to target the abnormal cells, killing them or inhibiting growth. Unlike chemo there are no known adverse side effects. There is more research being done on this but, as a natural product and a citrus fruit it can't do any harm

A diet is surely never complete without fresh fruits and green vegetables, with individuals being much more health aware. The oranges, carrots along with the banana are an essential section of the routine, healthful diet. It's high time we uncovered what soursop can do to your health. The leaves can be used as herbs for treating different ailments. The seeds which have emetic properties certainly are a great combatant fighting against nausea and vomiting. By mashing and mixing the leaves right into a concoction, apply it to the entire scalp and head lice can be reduced by you and reinforce the origins of the locks. If you're suffering from the wound, the fresh, crushed leaves can do wonders for a treatment for natural healing. People that have eczema can use mashed leaves as poultice so your skin issues could be relieved. Regularly you feel just like gulping juice rather than mastication the fruit, if the requirement add fresh fruits within our diet is improving with each passing day. If you ingestion the juice, it helps in treating liver troubles.

Do you think Cancer Be Healed With Soursop Fruit?

When talking about <u>soursop and cancer</u> cure, Soursop can be said to have some incredible skill when it comes to battling out the fatal disorder, cancer. According to researches that were carried out, which reveal it is quite powerful when it comes to slowing down the speed of cancer cells more compared to classic chemotherapy drugs.

Reference:

https://www.amazon.com/dp/B00PCPOHK2

www.ingramcontent.com/pod-product-compliance
Lightning Source LLC
Chambersburg PA
CBHW060826290526
45792CB00005BB/1813